Ketogenic Air Fryer Delights

Get in Shape and Lose Weight with Tasty and Affordable Recipes for Beginners

Chris Morgan

advice. The content within this book has been derived from various sources. Please consult a licensed professional before attempting any techniques outlined in this book.

By reading this document, the reader agrees that under no circumstances is the author responsible for any losses, direct or indirect, which are incurred as a result of the use of information contained within this document, including, but not limited to, — errors, omissions, or inaccuracies.

Table of Contents

Oregano and Lemon Chicken Drumsticks

Prep time: 15 minutes

Cooking time: 21 minutes

Servings: 4

Ingredients:

4 chicken drumsticks, with skin, bone-in

1 teaspoon dried cilantro

½ teaspoon dried oregano

½ teaspoon salt

1 teaspoon lemon juice

1 teaspoon butter, softened

2 garlic cloves, diced

Directions:

In the mixing bowl mix up dried cilantro, oregano, and salt. Then fill the chicken drumstick's skin with a cilantro mixture. Add butter and diced garlic. Sprinkle the chicken with lemon juice. Preheat the air fryer to 375F. Put the chicken drumsticks in the air fryer and cook them for 21 minutes.

Nutrition: calories 89, fat 3.6, fiber 0.1, carbs 0.7, protein 12.8

Thyme and Sage Turkey Breasts

Preparation time: 10 minutes

Cooking time: 25 minutes

Servings: 4

Ingredients:

turkey breasts, skinless, boneless and halved 4 tablespoons butter, melted

2 tablespoons thyme, chopped 2 tablespoons sage, chopped

tablespoons rosemary, chopped 2 tablespoons parsley, chopped A pinch of salt and black pepper 2 cups chicken stock

celery stalks, chopped

Directions:

Heat up a pan that fits your air fryer with the butter over medium-high heat, add the turkey and brown for 2-3 minutes on each side. Add the herbs, stock, celery, salt and pepper, toss, put the pan in your air fryer, cook at 390 degrees F for 20 minutes. Divide between plates and serve.

Nutrition: calories 284, fat 14, fiber 2, carbs 6, protein 20

Onion and Cayenne Chicken Tenders

Prep time: 15 minutes

Cooking time: 10 minutes

Servings: 2

Ingredients:

8 oz chicken fillet

1 teaspoon minced onion

¼ teaspoon onion powder

¼ teaspoon salt

½ teaspoon cayenne pepper

Cooking spray

Directions:

Cut the chicken fillet on 2 tenders and sprinkle with salt, onion powder, and cayenne pepper. Then preheat the air fryer to 365F. Spray the air fryer basket with cooking spray from inside and place the chicken tenders in it. Top the chicken with minced onion and cook for 10 minutes at 365F.

Nutrition: calories 219, fat 8.5, fiber 0.2, carbs 0.7, protein 32.9

Turkey and Butter Sauce

Preparation time: 5 minutes

Cooking time: 24 minutes

Servings: 4

Ingredients:

turkey breast, skinless, boneless and cut into 4 pieces A pinch of salt and black pepper

Juice of 1 lemon

tablespoons rosemary, chopped 2 tablespoons butter, melted

Directions:

In a bowl, mix the butter with the rosemary, lemon juice, salt and pepper and whisk really well. Brush the turkey pieces with the rosemary butter, put them your air fryer's basket, cook at 380 degrees F for 12 minutes on each side. Divide between plates and serve with a side salad.

Nutrition: calories 236, fat 12, fiber 4, carbs 6, protein 13

Garlic Chicken Sausages

Prep time: 20 minutes

Cooking time: 10 minutes

Servings: 4

Ingredients:

1 garlic clove, diced

1 spring onion, chopped

1 cup ground chicken

½ teaspoon salt

½ teaspoon ground black pepper

4 sausage links

1 teaspoon olive oil

Directions:

In the mixing bowl, mix up a diced garlic clove, onion, ground chicken, salt, and ground black pepper. Then fill the sausage links with the ground chicken mixture. Cut every sausage into halves and secure the endings.

Preheat the air fryer to 365. Brush the sausages with olive oil and put it in the air fryer. Cook them for 10 minutes. Then flip the sausages on another side and cook for 5 minutes more. Increase the Cooking time to 390F and cook for 8 minutes for faster results.

Nutrition: calories 130, fat 8.3, fiber 0.1, carbs 1, protein 12.2

Ginger Turkey and Cherry Tomatoes

Preparation time: 5 minutes

Cooking time: 25 minutes

Servings: 4

Ingredients:

pound turkey breast, skinless, boneless and cubed 1 cup heavy cream

A pinch of salt and black pepper 4 ounces cherry tomatoes, halved 1 tablespoon ginger, grated

tablespoons red chili powder 2 teaspoons olive oil

Directions:

Heat up a pan that fits the air fryer with the oil over medium heat, add the turkey and brown for 2 minutes on each side. Add the rest of the ingredients, toss, put the pan in the machine and cook at 380 degrees F for 20 minutes. Divide everything between plates and serve.

Nutrition: calories 267, fat 13, fiber 4, carbs 6, protein 16

Cayenne and Turmeric Chicken Strips

Prep time: 15 minutes

Cooking time: 14 minutes

Servings: 6

Ingredients:

2-pound chicken breast, skinless, boneless

1 teaspoon salt

1 teaspoon ground turmeric

½ teaspoon cayenne pepper

1 egg, beaten

2 tablespoons coconut flour

Directions:

Cut the chicken breast into the strips and sprinkle with salt, ground turmeric, and cayenne pepper. Then add beaten egg in the chicken strips and stir the mixture. After this, add coconut flour and stir it. Preheat the air fryer to 400F. Put ½ part of all chicken strips in the air fryer basket in one layer and cook them for 7 minutes. Repeat the same steps with the remaining chicken strips.

Nutrition: calories 195, fat 4.9, fiber 1, carbs 1.7, protein 33.4

Spiced Salmon and Cilantro Croquettes

Prep time: 10 minutes

Cooking time: 8 minutes

Servings: 4

Ingredients:

1-pound smoked salmon, boneless and flaked

1 egg, beaten

1 tablespoon almond flour

½ teaspoon ground black pepper

¼ teaspoon ground cumin

½ teaspoon ground nutmeg

1 tablespoon fresh cilantro, chopped

1 teaspoon avocado oil

Directions:

Put the salmon in the bowl and churn it with the help of the fork until you get the smooth mass. Then add an egg, almond flour, ground black pepper, cumin, nutmeg, and cilantro. Stir the ingredients until they are smooth. Preheat the air fryer to 365F. Wet your hands and make the croquettes. Then place them in the air fryer in one layer and sprinkle with avocado oil. Cook the croquettes for 5 minutes. Then flip them on another side and cook for 3 minutes more.

Nutrition: calories 210, fat 11.9, fiber 1, carbs 2, protein 25

Oregano Cod and Arugula Mix

Preparation time: 5 minutes

Cooking time: 12 minutes

Servings: 4

Ingredients:

tablespoons fresh cilantro, minced

pound cod fillets, boneless, skinless and cubed 1 spring onion, chopped

Salt and black pepper to the taste

½ teaspoon sweet paprika

½ teaspoon oregano, ground A drizzle of olive oil

cups baby arugula

Directions:

In a bowl, mix the cod with salt, pepper, paprika, oregano and the oil, toss, transfer the cubes to your air fryer's basket and cook at 360 degrees F for 12 minutes. In a salad bowl, mix the cod with the remaining ingredients, toss, divide between plates and serve.

Nutrition: calories 240, fat 11, fiber 3, carbs 5, protein 8

Shrimp Salad

Prep time: 15 minutes

Cooking time: 3 minutes

Servings: 4

Ingredients:

1-pound shrimps, peeled

1 tablespoon lemon juice

½ teaspoon ground cardamom

¼ teaspoon salt

½ teaspoon ground paprika

1 tablespoon olive oil

1 garlic clove, diced

1 avocado, peeled, pitted, chopped

1 teaspoon chives, chopped

Directions:

Put the shrimps in the big bowl. Add lemon juice, ground nutmeg, salt, and ground paprika. Mix up the shrimps and leave them for 10 minutes to marinate. Meanwhile, preheat the air fryer to 400F. Put the marinated shrimps in the air fryer and cook them for 3 minutes. It is recommended to arrange shrimps in one layer. Meanwhile, put the chopped avocado in the bowl and sprinkle it with diced garlic and chives. Cool the shrimps to the room temperature and add in the avocado bowl. Sprinkle the salad with olive oil. After this, gently mix the salad with the help of two spoons.

Nutrition: calories 271, fat 15.3, fiber 3.6, carbs 6.7, protein 26.9

Pork and Zucchinis

Preparation time: 5 minutes

Cooking time: 30 minutes

Servings: 4

Ingredients:

2 pounds pork stew meat, cubed 2 zucchinis, cubed

Salt and black pepper to the taste

½ cup beef stock

½ teaspoon smoked paprika A handful cilantro, chopped

Directions:

In a pan that fits your air fryer, mix all the ingredients, toss, introduce in your air fryer and cook at 370 degrees F for 30 minutes. Divide into bowls and serve right away.

Nutrition: calories 245, fat 12, fiber 2, carbs 5, protein 14

Rosemary Salmon

Prep time: 10 minutes

Cooking time: 7 minutes

Servings: 2

Ingredients:

4 oz Feta cheese, sliced

1 lemon slice, chopped

½ teaspoon dried rosemary

1 teaspoon apple cider vinegar

½ teaspoon ground paprika

1-pound salmon fillet

1 teaspoon olive oil

½ teaspoon salt

Cooking spray

Directions:

Rub the salmon with dried rosemary and salt. Then sprinkle the fish with ground paprika and apple cider vinegar. Preheat the air fryer to 395F. Line the air fryer basket with baking paper and put the salmon fillet on it. Spray it with cooking spray and cook for 3 minutes. Then flip the salmon on another side and cook it for 4 minutes more. After this, cut the cooked salmon into 2 servings and put it on the serving plate. Top the fish with sliced feta and chopped lemon slice. Sprinkle the meal with the olive oil before serving.

Nutrition: calories 596, fat 45, fiber 0.4, carbs 1.2, protein 47.4

Seafood Bowls

Preparation time: 5 minutes

Cooking time: 12 minutes

Servings: 4

Ingredients:

2 salmon fillets, boneless, skinless and cubed 8 ounces shrimp, peeled and deveined

Salt and black pepper to the taste 5 garlic cloves, minced teaspoon sweet paprika 2 tablespoons olive oil

Directions:

In a pan that fits the air fryer, combine all the ingredients, toss, cover and cook at 370 degrees F for 12 minutes. Divide into bowls and serve for lunch.

Nutrition: calories 270, fat 8, fiber 2, carbs 4, protein 7

Beef Chili

Prep time: 15 minutes

Cooking time: 29 minutes

Servings: 4

Ingredients:

2 spring onions, chopped

2 medium green bell peppers, chopped

1 tablespoon avocado oil

½ teaspoon salt

½ teaspoon ground black pepper

2 cups ground beef

1 teaspoon ground paprika

1 teaspoon chili flakes

½ teaspoon white pepper

1 teaspoon ground cumin

½ teaspoon ground coriander

1 chili pepper, chopped

1 cup beef broth

1 tablespoon keto tomato sauce

1 cup lettuce leaves

Directions:

Put the spring onions in the air fryer pan. Add green bell peppers, avocado oil, salt, and ground black pepper. Stir the mixture gently. Preheat the air fryer to 365F and place the pan with vegetables inside. Cook them for 4 minutes. Then stir well. In the mixing bowl mix up ground beef, ground paprika, chili flakes, white pepper, ground cumin, ground coriander, and tomato sauce Put the meat mixture over the vegetables and carefully stir it with the help of the spoon. Add chili pepper and beef broth. Stir the chili gently. Cook it at 365F for 25 minutes. Stir the chili every 5 minutes of cooking. When the chili is cooked, cool it for 5-10 minutes. Then fill the lettuce leaves with chili and transfer in the serving plates.

Nutrition: calories 177, fat 9.3, fiber 2.4, carbs 7.7, protein 15.5

Eggplant Bowls

Preparation time: 5 minutes

Cooking time: 15 minutes

Servings: 4

Ingredients:

cups eggplants, cubed 1 cup keto tomato sauce 1 teaspoon olive oil

1 cup mozzarella, shredded

Directions:

In a pan that fits the air fryer, combine all the ingredients except the mozzarella and toss. Sprinkle the cheese on top, introduce the pan in the machine and cook at 390 degrees F for 15 minutes. Divide between plates and serve for lunch.

Nutrition: calories 220, fat 9, fiber 2, carbs 6, protein 9

Chicken Rolls

Prep time: 15 minutes

Cooking time: 18 minutes

Servings: 4

Ingredients:

2 large zucchini

½ cup Cheddar cheese, shredded

1-pound chicken breast, skinless, boneless

1 teaspoon dried oregano

½ teaspoon olive oil

1 teaspoon salt

2 spring onions, chopped

1 teaspoon ground paprika

½ teaspoon ground turmeric

½ cup keto tomato sauce

Directions:

Preheat the skillet well and pour the olive oil inside. Put the onions in it and sprinkle with salt, ground paprika, and ground turmeric. Cook the onion for 5 minutes over the medium-high heat. Stir it from time to time. Meanwhile, shred the chicken. Add it in the skillet. Then add oregano. Stir well and cook the mixture for 2 minutes. After this, remove the skillet from the heat. Cut the zucchini into halves (lengthwise). Then make the zucchini slices with the help of the vegetable peeler. Put 3 zucchini slices on the chopping board overlapping each of them. Then spread the surface of them with the shredded chicken mixture. Roll the zucchini carefully in the shape of the roll. Repeat the same steps with remaining zucchini and shredded chicken mixture. Line the air fryer pan with parchment and put the enchilada rolls inside. Sprinkle them with tomato sauce Preheat the air fryer to 350F. Top the zucchini rolls (enchiladas) with Cheddar cheese and put in the air fryer basket. Cook the meal for 10 minutes.

Nutrition: calories 245, fat 9.3, fiber 3, carbs 10.3, protein 29.9

Chicken and Asparagus

Preparation time: 5 minutes

Cooking time: 20 minutes

Servings: 4

Ingredients:

4 chicken breasts, skinless, boneless and halved 1 tablespoon sweet paprika

bunch asparagus, trimmed and halved 1 tablespoon olive oil

Salt and black pepper to the taste

Directions:

In a bowl, mix all the ingredients, toss, put them in your Air Fryer's basket and cook at 390 degrees F for 20 minutes. Divide between plates and serve for lunch.

Nutrition: calories 230, fat 11, fiber 3, carbs 5, protein 12

Tarragon Sea Bass and Risotto

Preparation time: 5 minutes

Cooking time: 25 minutes

Servings: 4

Ingredients:

4 sea bass fillets, boneless

A pinch of salt and black pepper 1 tablespoon ghee, melted

1 garlic clove, minced 1 cup cauliflower rice

½ cup chicken stock

1 tablespoon parmesan, grated 1 tablespoon chervil, chopped 1 tablespoon parsley, chopped 1 tablespoon tarragon, chopped

Directions:

In a pan that fits your air fryer, mix the cauliflower rice with the stock, parmesan, chervil, tarragon and parsley, toss, introduce the pan in the air fryer and cook at 380 degrees F for 12 minutes. In a bowl, mix the fish with salt, pepper, garlic and melted ghee and toss gently. Put the fish over the cauliflower rice, cook at 380 degrees F for 12 minutes more, divide everything between plates and serve.

Nutrition: calories 261, fat 12, fiber 4, carbs 6, protein 11

Taco Lobster

Prep time: 10 minutes

Cooking time: 6 minutes

Servings: 4

Ingredients:

4 lettuce leaves

½ teaspoon taco seasonings

4 lobster tails

1 teaspoon Splenda

½ teaspoon ground cumin

½ teaspoon chili flakes

1 tablespoon ricotta cheese

1 teaspoon avocado oil

Directions:

Peel the lobster tails and sprinkle with ground cumin, taco seasonings, and chili flakes. Arrange the lobster tails in the air fryer basket and sprinkle with avocado oil. Cook them for 6 minutes at 380F. After this, remove the cooked lobster tails from the air fryer and chop them roughly. Transfer the lobster tails into the bowl. Add ricotta cheese and Splenda. Mix them up. Place the lobster mixture on the lettuce leaves and fold them.

Nutrition: calories 92, fat 1.2, fiber 0.1, carbs 2.1, protein 16.7

Peppercorn Cod

Preparation time: 5 minutes

Cooking time: 15 minutes

Servings: 4

Ingredients:

4 cod fillets, boneless

A pinch of salt and black pepper 1 tablespoon thyme, chopped

½ teaspoon black peppercorns 2 tablespoons olive oil

fennel, sliced

garlic cloves, minced

red bell pepper, chopped

teaspoons Italian seasoning

Directions:

In a bowl, mix the fennel with bell pepper and the other ingredients except the fish fillets and toss. Put this into a pan that fits the air fryer, add the fish on top, introduce the pan in your air fryer and cook at 380 degrees F for 15 minutes. Divide between plates and serve.

Nutrition: calories 241, fat 12, fiber 4, carbs 7, protein 11

Creamy Cod Strips

Prep time: 10 minutes

Cooking time: 6 minutes

Servings: 4

Ingredients:

10 oz cod fillet

1 tablespoon coconut flour

1 tablespoon coconut flakes

1 egg, beaten

1 teaspoon ground turmeric

½ teaspoon salt

1 tablespoon heavy cream

1 teaspoon olive oil

Directions:

Cut the cod fillets on the fries strips. After this, in the mixing bowl mix up coconut flour, coconut flakes, ground turmeric, and salt. In the other bowl mix up egg and heavy cream. After this, dip the fish fries in the egg mixture. Then coat them in the coconut flour mixture. Repeat the steps again. Preheat the air fryer to 400F. Put the fish fries in the air fryer basket in one layer and sprinkle them with olive oil. Cook the meal for 3 minutes. Then flip the fish fries on another side and cook for 3 minutes more.

Nutrition: calories 111, fat 5.1, fiber 1, carbs 1.9, protein 14.6

Chili Sea Bass Mix

Preparation time: 5 minutes

Cooking time: 15 minutes

Servings: 4

Ingredients:

4 sea bass fillets, boneless 4 garlic cloves, minced Juice of 1 lime

1 cup veggie stock

A pinch of salt and black pepper

1 tablespoon black peppercorns, crushed 1-inch ginger, grated

4 lemongrass, chopped 4 small chilies, minced

bunch coriander, chopped

Directions:

In a blender, combine all the ingredients except the fish and pulse well. Pour the mix in a pan that fits the air fryer, add the fish, toss, introduce in the fryer and cook at 380 degrees F for 15 minutes. Divide between plates and serve.

Nutrition: calories 271, fat 12, fiber 4, carbs 6, protein 12

Buttery Haddock and Parsley

Prep time: 10 minutes

Cooking time: 16 minutes

Servings: 2

Ingredients:

7 oz haddock fillet

2 tablespoons butter, melted

1 teaspoon minced garlic

½ teaspoon salt

1 teaspoon fresh parsley, chopped

½ teaspoon ground celery root

Directions:

Cut the fish fillet on 2 servings. In the shallow bowl mix up butter and minced garlic. Then add salt, celery root, and fresh parsley. After this, carefully brush the fish fillets with the butter mixture. Then wrap every fillet in the foil. Preheat the air fryer to 385F. Put the wrapped haddock fillets in the air fryer and cook for 16 minutes.

Nutrition: calories 215, fat 12.5, fiber 0.1, carbs 0.5, protein 24.3

Italian Shrimp Bowls

Preparation time: 5 minutes

Cooking time: 10 minutes

Servings: 4

Ingredients:

pounds shrimp, peeled and deveined A drizzle of olive oil

¼ cup chicken stock

1 tablespoon Italian seasoning Salt and black pepper to the taste

1 teaspoon red pepper flakes, crushed 8 garlic cloves, crushed

Directions:

Grease a pan that fits your air fryer with the oil, add the shrimp and the rest of the ingredients, toss, introduce the pan in the fryer and cook at 390 degrees F for 10 minutes. Divide into bowls and serve.

Nutrition: calories 261, fat 12, fiber 6, carbs 7, protein 12

Tarragon and Spring Onions Salmon

Prep time: 15 minutes

Cooking time: 15 minutes

Servings: 4

Ingredients:

12 oz salmon fillet

2 spring onions, chopped

1 tablespoon ghee, melted

1 teaspoon peppercorns

½ teaspoon salt

½ teaspoon ground black pepper

1 teaspoon tarragon

½ teaspoon dried cilantro

Directions:

Cut the salmon fillet on 4 servings. Then make the parchment pockets and place the fish fillets in the parchment pockets. Sprinkle the salmon with salt, ground black pepper, tarragon, and dried cilantro. After this, top the fish with spring onions, peppercorns, and ghee. Preheat the air fryer to 385F. Arrange the salmon pockets in the air fryer in one layer and cook them for 15 minutes.

Nutrition: calories 154, fat 8.5, fiber 0.8, carbs 3.2, protein 16.9

Shrimp and Scallions

Preparation time: 3 minutes

Cooking time: 10 minutes

Servings: 4

Ingredients:

1 pound shrimp, peeled and deveined 2 tablespoons olive oil

1 tablespoon scallions, chopped 1 cup chicken stock

Directions:

In a pan that fits your air fryer, mix the shrimp with the oil, onion and the stock, introduce the pan in the fryer and cook at 380 degrees F for 10 minutes. Divide into bowls and serve.

Nutrition: calories 261, fat 6, fiber 8, carbs 16, protein 6

Lemon Octopus

Prep time: 10 minutes

Cooking time: 26 minutes

Servings: 4

Ingredients:

11 oz octopus

1 teaspoon chili flakes

1 chili pepper, chopped

1 tablespoon coconut oil, melted

½ teaspoon salt

1 cup of water

1 tablespoon lemon juice

Directions:

Pour water in the pan and bring it to boil. Chop the octopus and put it in the boiling water. Close the lid and cook the seafood for 25 minutes. After this, remove the octopus from the water and sprinkle with chili flakes, chili pepper, coconut oil, salt, and lemon juice.

Transfer them in the air fryer and cook for 1 minute at 390F.

Nutrition: calories 159, fat 5.1, fiber 0.1, carbs 3.6, protein 23.3

Garlic Fish and Balsamic Salsa

Preparation time: 5 minutes

Cooking time: 15 minutes

Servings: 4

Ingredients:

4 sea bass fillets, boneless 1 tablespoon olive oil

3 tomatoes, roughly chopped 2 spring onions, chopped

¼ cup chicken stock

A pinch of salt and black pepper 3 garlic cloves, minced

1 tablespoon balsamic vinegar

Directions:

In a blender, combine all the ingredients except the fish and pulse well. Put the mix in a pan that fits the air fryer, add the fish, toss gently, introduce the pan in the fryer and cook at 380 degrees F for 15 minutes. Divide between plates and serve.

Nutrition: calories 261, fat 11, fiber 4, carbs 7, protein 11

French Clams

Prep time: 5 minutes

Cooking time: 3 minutes

Servings: 5

Ingredients:

2-pounds clams, raw, shells removed

1 tablespoon Herbs de Provence

1 tablespoon sesame oil

1 garlic clove, diced

Directions:

Put the clams in the bowl and sprinkle with Herbs de Provence, sesame oil, and diced garlic. Shake the seafood well. Preheat the air fryer to 390F. Put the clams in the air fryer and cook them for 3 minutes. When the clams are cooked, shake them well and transfer in the serving plates.

Nutrition: calories 45, fat 3, fiber 0, carbs 0.9, protein 3.5

Garlic Balsamic Tomatoes

Preparation time: 5 minutes

Cooking time: 15 minutes

Servings: 4

Ingredients:

1 tablespoon olive oil

1 pound cherry tomatoes, halved 1 tablespoon dill, chopped

6 garlic cloves, minced

1 tablespoon balsamic vinegar Salt and black pepper to the taste

Directions:

In a pan that fits the air fryer, combine all the ingredients, toss gently, put the pan in the air fryer and cook at 380 degrees F for 15 minutes. Divide between plates and serve.

Nutrition: calories 121, fat 3, fiber 2, carbs 4, protein 6

Almond Eggplant Meatballs

Prep time: 15 minutes

Cooking time: 8 minutes

Servings: 7

Ingredients:

3 eggplants, peeled, boiled

1 egg, beaten

1 teaspoon minced garlic

3 spring onions, chopped

½ cup almond flour

1 teaspoon chives

½ teaspoon chili flakes

½ teaspoon salt

1 teaspoon sesame oil

Directions:

Chop the boiled eggplants and squeeze the juice from them. After this, transfer the eggplants in the blender. Add egg, minced garlic, spring onions, almond flour, chives, chili flakes, and salt. Grind the mixture until it is homogenous and smooth. After this, make the eggplant meatballs from the mixture with the help of the scooper. Preheat the air fryer to 380F. Put the eggplant meatballs in the air fryer and sprinkle them with sesame oil. Cook the meatballs for 8 minutes.

Nutrition: calories 87, fat 2.7, fiber 8.6, carbs 14.8, protein 3.6

Cilantro Broccoli Mix

Preparation time: 5 minutes

Cooking time: 15 minutes

Servings: 4

Ingredients:

1 broccoli head, florets separated 2 cups cherry tomatoes, quartered A pinch of salt and black pepper 1 tablespoon cilantro, chopped Juice of 1 lime

A drizzle of olive oil

Directions:

In a pan that fits the air fryer, combine the broccoli with tomatoes and the rest of the ingredients except the cilantro, toss, put the pan in the air fryer and cook at 380 degrees F for 15 minutes. Divide between plates and serve with cilantro sprinkled on top.

Nutrition: calories 141, fat 3, fiber 2, carbs 4, protein 5

Mustard Cabbage

Prep time: 10 minutes

Cooking time: 40 minutes

Servings: 4

Ingredients:

1-pound white cabbage

1 teaspoon mustard

1 teaspoon ground black pepper

½ teaspoon salt

3 tablespoons butter, melted

½ teaspoon ground paprika

½ teaspoon chili flakes

1 teaspoon dried thyme

Directions:

In the mixing bowl mix up mustard, ground black pepper, salt, butter, ground paprika, chili flakes, and dried thyme. Brush the cabbage with the mustard mixture generously and place it in the air fryer. Cook the cabbage for 40 minutes at 365F. Then cool the cooked vegetable to the room temperature and slice into servings.

Nutrition: calories 111, fat 9.1, fiber 3.3, carbs 7.5, protein 1.9

Cajun Zucchini and Broccoli

Prep time: 10 minutes

Cooking time: 15 minutes

Servings: 2

Ingredients:

½ zucchini, chopped

2 spring onions, chopped

¼ cup broccoli, chopped

1 teaspoon Cajun seasonings

1 teaspoon nut oil

2 oz fennel bulb, chopped

Directions:

In the mixing bowl mix up all ingredients. Then preheat the air fryer to 385F. Put the mixture in the air fryer and cook it for 15 minutes. Shake the vegetables every 5 minutes.

Nutrition: calories 46, fat 2.5, fiber 2, carbs 5.8, protein 1.4

Lime Olives and Zucchini

Preparation time: 5 minutes

Cooking time: 12 minutes

Servings: 4

Ingredients:

4 zucchinis, sliced

cup kalamata olives, pitted Salt and black pepper to the taste 2 tablespoons lime juice

tablespoons olive oil

2 teaspoons balsamic vinegar

Directions:

In a pan that fits your air fryer, mix the olives with all the other ingredients, toss, introduce in the fryer and cook at 390 degrees F for 12 minutes. Divide the mix between plates and serve.

Nutrition: calories 150, fat 4, fiber 2, carbs 4, protein 5

Cream Cheese Green Beans

Prep time: 15 minutes

Cooking time: 5 minutes

Servings: 2

Ingredients:

8 oz green beans

1 egg, beaten

1 teaspoon cream cheese

¼ cup almond flour

¼ cup coconut flakes

½ teaspoon ground black pepper

½ teaspoon salt

1 teaspoon sesame oil

Directions:

In the mixing bowl mix up cream cheese, egg, and ground black pepper. Add salt. In the separated bowl mix up coconut flakes and almond flour. Preheat the air fryer to 400F. Dip the green beans in the egg mixture and then coat in the coconut flakes mixture. Repeat the step one more time and transfer the vegetables in the air fryer. Sprinkle them with sesame oil and cook for 5 minutes. Shake the vegetables after 2 minutes of cooking if you don't put green beans in one layer.

Nutrition: calories 149, fat 10.3, fiber 5.3, carbs 10.9, protein 6.1

Tomato Artichokes Mix

Preparation time: 5 minutes

Cooking time: 15 minutes

Servings: 4

Ingredients:

14 ounces artichoke hearts, drained 1 tablespoon olive oil

2 cups black olives, pitted 3 garlic cloves, minced

½ cup keto tomato sauce 1 teaspoon garlic powder

Directions:

In a pan that fits your air fryer, mix the olives with the artichokes and the other ingredients, toss, put the pan in the fryer and cook at 350 degrees F for 15 minutes. Divide the mix between plates and serve.

Nutrition: calories 180, fat 4, fiber 3, carbs 5, protein 6

Taco Okra

Prep time: 10 minutes

Cooking time: 10 minutes

Servings: 3

Ingredients:

9 oz okra, chopped

1 teaspoon taco seasoning

1 teaspoon sunflower oil

Directions:

In the mixing bowl mix up chopped okra, taco seasoning, and sunflower oil. Then preheat the air fryer to 385F. Put the okra mixture in the air fryer and cook it for 5 minutes. Then shake the vegetables well and cook them for 5 minutes more.

Nutrition: calories 51, fat 1.7, fiber 2.7, carbs 7, protein 1.6

Spicy Olives and Tomato Mix

Preparation time: 5 minutes

Cooking time: 15 minutes

Servings: 4

Ingredients:

2 cups kalamata olives, pitted

2 small avocados, pitted, peeled and sliced

¼ cup cherry tomatoes, halved Juice of 1 lime

1 tablespoon coconut oil, melted

Directions:

In a pan that fits the air fryer, combine the olives with the other ingredients, toss, put the pan in your air fryer and cook at 370 degrees F for 15 minutes. Divide the mix between plates and serve.

Nutrition: calories 153, fat 3, fiber 3, carbs 4, protein 6

Baked Plum Cream

Preparation time: 5 minutes

Cooking time: 20 minutes

Servings: 4

Ingredients:

1 pound plums, pitted and chopped

¼ cup swerve

tablespoon lemon juice 1 and ½ cups heavy cream

Directions:

In a bowl, mix all the ingredients and whisk really well. Divide this into 4 ramekins, put them in the air fryer and cook at 340 degrees F for 20 minutes. Serve cold.

Nutrition: calories 171, fat 4, fiber 2, carbs 4, protein 4

Vinegar Cake

Prep time: 25 minutes

Cooking time: 30 minutes

Servings: 4

Ingredients:

2 teaspoons cream cheese

1 teaspoon Truvia

1 teaspoon vanilla extract

½ cup heavy cream

1 egg, beaten

1 teaspoon baking powder

1 teaspoon apple cider vinegar

1 ½ cup coconut flour

2 tablespoons butter, softened

Cooking spray

Directions:

Pour heavy cream in the bowl. Add vanilla extract, egg, baking powder, apple cider vinegar, and butter. Stir the liquid until homogenous. Then add coconut flour. Whisk the liquid until smooth. Spray the pound cake mold with cooking spray. Pour the pound cake batter in the mold. Flatten its surface with the help of the spatula. Preheat the air fryer to 365F. Put the mold with the pound cake in the air fryer and cook it for 30 minutes.

When the cake is cooked, cool it to the room temperature. Meanwhile, in the shallow bowl whisk together cream cheese and Truvia. Then spread the surface of the pound cake with sweet cream cheese. Slice the dessert on the servings.

Nutrition: calories 339, fat 20.5, fiber 18, carbs 28.7, protein 10.9

Blackberries Cake

Preparation time: 10 minutes

Cooking time: 25 minutes

Servings: 4

Ingredients:

eggs, whisked

4 tablespoons swerve

2 tablespoons ghee, melted

¼ cup almond milk

1 and ½ cups almond flour 1 cup blackberries, chopped

½ teaspoon baking powder

teaspoon lemon zest, grated 1 teaspoon lemon juice

Directions:

In a bowl, mix all the ingredients and whisk well. Pour this into a cake pan that fits the air fryer lined with parchment paper, put the pan in your air fryer and cook at 340 degrees F for 25 minutes. Cool the cake down, slice and serve.

Nutrition: calories 193, fat 5, fiber 1, carbs 4, protein 4

Cardamom Coconut Cookies

Prep time: 15 minutes

Cooking time: 10 minutes

Servings: 6

Ingredients:

3 tablespoons coconut oil, softened

4 tablespoons coconut flour

2 tablespoons flax meal

2 tablespoons Monk fruit

1 teaspoon poppy seeds

½ teaspoon baking powder

½ teaspoon lemon juice

¼ teaspoon ground cardamom

Cooking spray

Directions:

In the mixing bowl put coconut oil, coconut flour, flax meal, ad Monk fruit. Then add poppy seeds, baking powder, lemon juice, and cardamom. With the help of the fingertips knead the soft but non-sticky dough. Then make the cookies from the dough. Preheat the air fryer to 375F. Spray the air fryer basket with cooking spray. Place the cookies in the air fryer and cook them for 10 minutes.

Nutrition: calories 95, fat 8.7, fiber 2.8, carbs 4, protein 1.6

Butter Plums

Preparation time: 5 minutes

Cooking time: 20 minutes

Servings: 4

Ingredients:

teaspoons cinnamon powder 4 plums, halved

4 tablespoons butter, melted 3 tablespoons swerve

Directions:

In a pan that fits your air fryer, mix the plums with the rest of the ingredients, toss, put the pan in the air fryer and cook at 300 degrees F for 20 minutes. Divide into cups and serve cold.

Nutrition: calories 162, fat 3, fiber 2, carbs 4, protein 5

Nuts Cookie s

Prep time: 15 minutes

Cooking time: 10 minutes

Servings: 6

Ingredients:

½ cup butter, softened

1 cup coconut flour

3 oz macadamia nuts, grinded

½ teaspoon baking powder

3 tablespoons Erythritol

Cooking spray

Directions:

In the mixing bowl mix up butter, coconut flour, grinded coconut nuts, baking powder, and Erythritol. Knead the non-sticky dough. Cut the dough into small pieces and roll them into balls. Press every cookie ball gently to get the shape of cookies. Preheat the air fryer to 365F. Spray the air fryer basket with cooking spray. Put the uncooked cookies in the air fryer and cook them for 8 minutes. Then cook for extra 2 minutes at 390F to get the light brown crust.

Nutrition: calories 331, fat 29.4, fiber 9.2, carbs 14.2, protein 5.3

Lemon Berries Stew

Preparation time: 10 minutes

Cooking time: 20 minutes

Servings: 4

Ingredients:

1 pound strawberries, halved 4 tablespoons stevia

tablespoon lemon juice 1 and ½ cups water

Directions:

In a pan that fits your air fryer, mix all the ingredients, toss, put it in the fryer and cook at 340 degrees F for 20 minutes. Divide the stew into cups and serve cold.

Nutrition: calories 176, fat 2, fiber 1, carbs 3, protein 5

Whipped Cream Cake

Prep time: 15 minutes

Cooking time: 25 minutes

Servings: 12

Ingredients:

1 cup almond flour

½ cup coconut flour

¼ cup coconut oil, melted

3 eggs, beaten

1 teaspoon baking powder

1 teaspoon vanilla extract

1 teaspoon cream cheese

2 tablespoons Splenda

½ cup whipped cream

Directions:

In the mixing bowl mix up almond flour, coconut flour, coconut oil, eggs, baking powder, vanilla extract, and cream cheese. Whisk the mixture well with the help of the immersion blender. Then line the air fryer baking pan with baking paper. Pour the cake batter in the baking pan. Preheat the air fryer to 355F. Put the baking pan in the air fryer and cook it for 25 minutes. Then cool the cake well. Meanwhile, mix up Splenda and whipped cream cheese. Spread the cake with whipped cream mixture.

Nutrition: calories 119, fat 9.3, fiber 2.3, carbs 6, protein 3

Chocolate and Avocado Cream

Preparation time: 5 minutes

Cooking time: 20 minutes

Servings: 4

Ingredients:

avocados, peeled, pitted and mashed 3 tablespoons chocolate, melted

4 tablespoons erythritol

3 tablespoons cream cheese, soft

Directions:

In a pan that fits the air fryer, combine all the ingredients, whisk, put the pan in the fryer and cook at 340 degrees F for 20 minutes. Divide into bowls and serve cold.

Nutrition: calories 200, fat 6, fiber 2, carbs 4, protein 5

Sweet Coconut Cream Pie

Prep time: 15 minutes

Cooking time: 25 minutes

Servings: 4

Ingredients:

4 tablespoons coconut cream

1 teaspoon baking powder

1 teaspoon apple cider vinegar

1 egg, beaten

¼ cup coconut flakes

1 teaspoon vanilla extract

½ cup coconut flour

4 teaspoons Splenda

1 teaspoon xanthan gum

Cooking spray

Directions:

Put all liquid ingredients in the bowl: coconut cream, apple cider vinegar, egg, and vanilla extract. Stir the liquid until homogenous and add baking powder, coconut flakes, coconut flour, Splenda, and xanthan gum. Stir the ingredients until you get the smooth texture of the batter. Spray the air fryer cake mold with cooking spray. Pour the batter in the cake mold.

Preheat the air fryer to 330F. Put the cake mold in the air fryer basket and cook it for 25 minutes. Then cool the cooked pie completely and remove it from the cake mold. Cut the cooked pie into servings.

Nutrition: calories 110, fat 6.6, fiber 3.9, carbs 9.9, protein 2.1

Cocoa Bombs

Preparation time: 5 minutes

Cooking time: 8 minutes

Servings: 12

Ingredients:

2 cups macadamia nuts, chopped 4 tablespoons coconut oil, melted 1 teaspoon vanilla extract

¼ cup cocoa powder 1/3 cup swerve

Directions:

In a bowl, mix all the ingredients and whisk well. Shape medium balls out of this mix, place them in your air fryer and cook at 300 degrees F for 8 minutes. Serve cold.

Nutrition: calories 120, fat 12, fiber 1, carbs 2, protein 1

Cinnamon Squash Pie

Prep time: 15 minutes

Cooking time: 35 minutes

Servings: 6

Ingredients:

2 tablespoons Splenda

1 tablespoon Erythritol

5 eggs, beaten

4 tablespoons coconut flakes

¼ cup heavy cream

1 teaspoon vanilla extract

1 teaspoon butter

¼ teaspoon ground cinnamon

4 oz Kabocha squash, peeled

Directions:

Grate the Kabocha squash. Then grease the baking mold with butter and put the grated Kabocha squash inside. In the mixing bowl mix up Splenda, Erythritol, coconut flakes, heavy cream, vanilla extract, and ground cinnamon. Then pour the liquid over the Kabocha squash. Stir the mixture gently with the help of the fork. Then preheat the air fryer to 365F. Put the mold with pie in the air fryer and cook it for 35 minutes. Cool the cooked pie to the room temperature and cut into the servings.

Nutrition: calories 116, fat 7.2, fiber 0.6, carbs 6.7, protein 5.1

Avocado Cake

Preparation time: 10 minutes

Cooking time: 30 minutes

Servings: 4

Ingredients:

4 ounces raspberries

avocados, peeled, pitted and mashed 1 cup almonds flour

teaspoons baking powder 1 cup swerve

tablespoons butter, melted 4 eggs, whisked

Directions:

In a bowl, mix all the ingredients, toss, pour this into a cake pan that fits the air fryer after you've lined it with parchment paper, put the pan in the fryer and cook at 340 degrees F for 30 minutes. Leave the cake to cool down, slice and serve.

Nutrition: calories 193, fat 4, fiber 2, carbs 5, protein 5

Blueberry Cookies

Prep time: 10 minutes

Cooking time: 30 minutes

Servings: 2

Ingredients:

3 oz blueberries

½ teaspoon avocado oil

Directions:

Put the blueberries in the blender and grind them until smooth. Then line the air fryer basket with baking paper. Brush it with the avocado oil. After this, pour the blended blueberries on the prepared baking paper and flatten it in one layer with the help of the spatula. Cook the blueberry leather for 30 minutes at 300F. Cut into cookies and serve.

Nutrition: calories 26, fat 0.3, fiber 1.1, carbs 6.2, protein 0.3

Cinnamon and Butter Pancakes

Prep time: 10 minutes

Cooking time: 12 minutes

Servings: 2

Ingredients:

1 teaspoon ground cinnamon

2 teaspoons butter, softened

1 teaspoon baking powder

½ teaspoon lemon juice

½ teaspoon vanilla extract

¼ cup heavy cream

4 tablespoons almond flour

2 teaspoons Erythritol

Directions:

Preheat the air fryer to 325F. Take 2 small cake mold and line them with baking paper. After this, in the mixing bowl mix up ground cinnamon, butter, baking powder, lemon juice, vanilla extract, heavy cream, almond flour, and Erythritol. Stir the mixture until it is smooth. Then pour the mixture in the prepared cake molds. Put the first cake mold in the air fryer and cook the pancake for 6 minutes. Then check if the pancake is cooked (it should have light brown color) and remove it from the air fryer. Repeat the same steps with the second pancake. It is recommended to serve the pancakes warm or hot.

Nutrition: calories 414, fat 37.4, fiber 6.7, carbs 14.7, protein 12.4

Strawberry Cups

Preparation time: 5 minutes

Cooking time: 10 minutes

Servings: 8

Ingredients:

16 strawberries, halved

2 tablespoons coconut oil

2 cups chocolate chips, melted

Directions:

In a pan that fits your air fryer, mix the strawberries with the oil and the melted chocolate chips, toss gently, put the pan in the air fryer and cook at 340 degrees F for 10 minutes. Divide into cups and serve cold.

Nutrition: calories 162, fat 5, fiber 3, carbs 5, protein 6

Cardamom Squares

Prep time: 15 minutes

Cooking time: 20 minutes

Servings: 4

Ingredients:

4 tablespoons peanut butter

1 tablespoon peanut, chopped

1 teaspoon vanilla extract

½ cup coconut flour

1 tablespoon Erythritol

½ teaspoon ground cardamom

Directions:

Put the peanut butter and peanut in the bowl. Add vanilla extract, coconut flour, and ground cardamom. Then add Erythritol and stir the mixture until homogenous. Preheat the air fryer to 330F. Line the air fryer basket with baking paper and pour the peanut butter mixture over it. Flatten it gently and cook for 20 minutes. Then remove the cooked mixture from the air fryer and cool it completely. Cut the dessert into the squares.

Nutrition: calories 181, fat 11.7, fiber 7.2, carbs 12.8, protein 7.6

Strawberry Cake

Preparation time: **10 minutes**

Cooking time: 35 minutes

Servings: 6

Ingredients:

1 pound strawberries, chopped 1 cup cream cheese, soft

¼ cup swerve

1 tablespoon lime juice 1 egg, whisked

1 teaspoon vanilla extract

3 tablespoons coconut oil, melted 1 cup almond flour

2 teaspoons baking powder

Directions:

In a bowl, mix all the ingredients, stir well and pour this into a cake pan lined with parchment paper. Put the pan in the air fryer, cook at 350 degrees F for 35 minutes, cool down, slice and serve.

Nutrition: calories 200, fat 6, fiber 2, carbs 4, protein 6

Chives and Lemon Chicken

Preparation time: 5 minutes

Cooking time: 20 minutes

Servings: 4

Ingredients:

1 pound chicken tenders, boneless, skinless A pinch of salt and black pepper

Juice of 1 lemon

tablespoon chives, chopped A drizzle of olive oil

Directions:

In a bowl, mix the chicken tenders with all ingredients except the chives, toss, put the meat in your air fryer's basket and cook at 370 degrees F for 10 minutes on each side. Divide between plates and serve with chives sprinkled on top.

Nutrition: calories 230, fat 13, fiber 4, carbs 6, protein 16

Sweet Turmeric Chicken Wings

Prep time: 15 minutes

Cooking time: 15 minutes

Servings: 8

Ingredients:

8 chicken wings

1 teaspoon Splenda

1 teaspoon ground turmeric

½ teaspoon cayenne pepper

1 tablespoon avocado oil

Directions:

Mix up Splenda and avocado oil and stir the mixture until Splenda is dissolved. Then rub the chicken wings with ground turmeric and cayenne pepper. Brush the chicken wings with sweet avocado oil from both sides. Preheat the air fryer to 390F. Place the chicken wings in the air fryer and cook them for 15 minutes.

Nutrition: calories 105, fat 6.9, fiber 0.2, carbs 0.8, protein 9.2

Red Vinegar and Chicken Mix

Preparation time: 5 minutes

Cooking time: 30 minutes

Servings: 4

Ingredients:

pounds chicken wings, halved

¼ cup red vinegar

4 garlic cloves, minced

Salt and black pepper to the taste 4 tablespoons olive oil

tablespoon garlic powder 1 teaspoon turmeric powder

Directions:

In a bowl, mix the chicken with all the other ingredients and toss well. Put the chicken wings in your air fryer's basket and cook at 370 degrees F for 30 minutes, flipping the meat halfway. Divide everything between plates and serve with a side salad.

Nutrition: calories 250, fat 12, fiber 4, carbs 6, protein 15

Lightning Source UK Ltd.
Milton Keynes UK
UKHW020645290621
386332UK00001B/35

9 781803 423647